WEIGHT LOSS FOR LIFE FOR REGULAR PEOPLE

WEIGHT LOSS FOR LIFE FOR REGULAR PEOPLE

Robin Baines MD

ISBN 9781792399350

For additional information email

Allaboutyouwellness.net@gmail.com

In dedication to all of us who try daily
to be our healthiest version.

Table of Contents

Introduction ix

Chapter 1 What Is Your Why? 1

Chapter 2 You Did Not Fail 5

Chapter 3 Your Ideal Weight 10

Chapter 4 You've Got To Eat Something! 15

Chapter 5 Who Has Time For That? 25

Chapter 6 Have A Notion For Motion 30

Chapter 7 How Do You Use Food? 37

Chapter 8 Planning is Everything 41

Chapter 9 Stress Less And Rest Well 45

Chapter 10 Food Addiction 49

Chapter 11 What Has Worked For Others? 53

Conclusion 56

Introduction

We understand the many benefits and importance of maintaining a healthy weight. However, achieving long lasting results seems to be a never-ending pursuit. So much information is available and yet the problem persists. Diets, pills, exercise and no lasting outcomes causes frustration when there's nothing to show for all the effort.

What you learn in this book will help you to attain weight loss in practical ways. By the end you will:

1. understand why you want to lose weight

2. identify past successes and opportunities to improve on your weight loss efforts for long-term success

3. determine what you want to accomplish and how you will track your progress

4. identify possible impediments to your success

5. appreciate the value of movement

6. understand how to make healthful food choices

7. understand the role stress and sleep play in weight management

You will not find magic potions, super food pill recommendations, push for supplements, specific meal plans or other extremes here. Reading this book does not guarantee a certain number of pounds will be lost in a certain period of time. No gimmicks. *Weight Loss*

For Life For Regular People offers you data, facts and recommendations for weight loss choices that support a healthy life.

Take your time with this material. Sit with the information you are learning. Take time to process and think about how you can apply what you're learning. Be true to yourself and be realistic. You may find you need to read a chapter multiple times or even read the chapters in a different order. Do whatever you need to digest the material and make it work for you.

As you identify your own strengths, weakness and opportunities and implement what you are learning you will improve your life proportional to your effort.

Chapter 1

What Is Your Why?

It's always helpful to start with "why." Your why will direct your path. It will provoke more questions and considerations. It will make you balance and reconsider. It will help you to see and focus on the big picture. Stephen Covey puts it this way, "begin with the end in mind." Your why and where it takes you is powerful.

Why do you want to lose weight?

What will weight loss mean for you?

Will it prove something to yourself or someone else?

Will you be a "better person" and if so, how?

Will it increase your confidence?

Something else?

What will you do as a thinner person that differs from what you do now?

Will it improve your agility?

Will less of you (i.e. weight) make you feel more visible?

Something else?

What opportunities and options will weight loss afford you?

Will it increase your pool of people to date?

Will it position you for higher income?

Something else?

What if you do not lose weight?

Will you benefit from the process if you don't accomplish your goal?

How does your future look at your current weight?

Something else?

What do you have to lose?

Do you find comfort in your weight?

Is your weight a large part of your identity?

Something else?

What do you have to gain?

How could your future look as a thinner person?

Will weight loss position you for success?

Something else?

Questions, Questions, Questions

These questions are everything. Changing your lifestyle is HUGE and not for the faint of heart. It requires significant mental and emotional energy. It takes effort and foresight. Your current lifestyle is what you've created, but it did not happen overnight. It has been a lifetime in the making. How much do you want to tweak it? They say, "don't mess with perfection" right? After all, you have made it this far! Is it worth it to change?

Answers, Answers, Answers

The answers must be compelling enough to push you pass all impediments. They need only make sense to you. They should propel you to the next level. And guess what? You define the next level. **Your** why is **your** motivation.

All About You

The answers to the questions are personal. Only you need to understand your "why." The answers vary from person to person, job to job, culture to culture. We all have different reasons. For some it is general health, a personal health goal like reducing medications, appearance, energy, family member's health, impact on family, etc. The potential reasons are numerous but none of them matter if it is not your own "why." At the end of the day you are all you actually have, own and control. Your answers should be applicable regardless of your setting, work place, state you live in, clubs you belong to, etc. Your answers are personal based on your own goals for yourself.

Consideration to get you thinking:

1. What is my why?

Chapter 2

You Did Not Fail

Many people feel they have failed in their attempts to lose and maintain weight loss. Actually, you have responded normally, given how we live. Weight loss is **not just a matter of willpower**.

Excess body weight is not:

A sign of low vigor or stamina

A sign of laziness

A sign of low ambition

A lack of care

Excess body weight is an expected response to the environment we've created. Willpower is great, but it's not enough. It helps when you need an occasional boost but not for a daily lifestyle change. Willpower runs out.

The truth is losing weight and keeping it off is forcing the body to do something it is not designed to do. Evolutionarily speaking, excess body fat would have been protective in times of deprivation when food and food sources were not readily available. Excess body fat in that setting would have supported longer survival due to more stored energy. So it can be a fight and definite challenge to overcome the body's innate drives and tendencies. Some approaches just do not support sustained weight loss.

Hunger, eating and feeling full is really a very complicated process. So many signals in our bodies are at play at any given time. The digestive tract is in communication with the brain to turn on eating with signals like- neuropeptide y, melanin concentrating hormone, orexin, galanin, agouti related protein and ghrelin to name some that we are familiar with. The digestive tract communicates with the brain to stop eating with signals like serotonin, peptide yy, alpha melanocyte stimulating hormone and amylin to name some. We also now know that fat tissue is active, not just stored energy. It secretes a hormone signal called leptin that communicates with the brain. My point is getting hunger, eating and fullness right for a healthy weight is very complex. None of the above signals are changed by the strongest willpower.

There are so many contributors to excess body fat. Some medications contribute like migraine preventatives, hypnotics, mood stabilizers, anti-seizure medications, steroids, antipsychotics, antidepressant and insulin to name some. Some medical problems cause weight gain like hypothyroidism and Cushing Syndrome. Some mental health problem like depression and anxiety can impact weight. These problems can be controlled and treated.

Genetics can play a role. However, this is not a significant contribution for most. <10% of obesity is related to a genetic problem. We may inherit genetic predisposition with regard to how our bodies handle calories, store calories and energy for activity. However, genetic predisposition means the back ground exists for potential problems. Genetic predisposition does not mean a problem is destined to happen and is inevitable. Our life choices are much, much more powerful than our genetic predisposition.

Nutrition science now teaches us about the gut microbiome. The bacteria that live in our digestive tracts aide with digestion, immune function and vitamin production. It turns out there are many more bacterial cells than human cells in the human body. The gut microbiome becomes populated with bacteria that promote or do not promote weight gain. Plant based high fiber foods support the growth of desirable bacteria. Animal products promote the growth of bacteria more associated with obesity.

Our modern environment contributes to our excess body fat. Very good tasting (i.e. highly palatable), high fat and high sugar (i.e. calorie dense) foods are abundant. These foods stimulate the reward center in the brain with dopamine release. We are inundated and targeted by commercials and in checkout lines. We are lured by the convenience of fast foods and packaged foods. Billboards grab our attention on our drive to work because we live too far to walk or cycle in our modern society. Our lifestyle and community are not conducive to physical activity with our lack of sidewalks and trails. We prefer the remote control to walking to the TV. Our conveniences are hurting us.

Our culture lends itself to indulgence, excess and efficiency. We see this as a sign of affluence and something to be desired. However, the more efficient we become, the less physically active we are and it parallels our hyper-consumption. We consume more of everything, not just food, but also entertainment and luxuries. Our socialization is punctuated by indulgent eating. We eat in sorrow after funerals and we eat in celebration for weddings, birthdays and graduations.

Obesogens, chemicals that contribute to obesity, are in our regular products. Examples of potential obesogens include:

Bisphenol- A (BPA) found in food containers and baby bottles

Phthalates used to make plastics soft and flexible

Perfluorooctanoic Acid (PFOA) found in nonstick cook ware

PCBs used in some lubricants

These are just a few that have had some study. There are many more known and under study.

You have not failed in your weight loss and weight loss maintenance attempts. You have had a normal response to this modern environment; however, you can do something about it.

Considerations to get you thinking:

1. How has my environment influenced my eating?

2. In what areas am I overly indulgent?

3. How will I begin to socialize without food?

Chapter 3

Your Ideal Weight

There are several measures to indicate body fatness. The most common is just weight. Body weight is made of more than just fat; it is also bones, muscles, water, etc. Body mass index takes it a step further by considering weight for height. Other measures are percent body fat, waist circumference, and waist to hip ratio. These measures can be calculated and measured at home. Ultimately it is body fat that is most relevant for most of us.

Body mass index (BMI) is calculated by measuring

$$\text{(Weight in pounds / height in inches /}$$
$$\text{height in inches)} \times 703$$

Weight in pounds, divided by height in inches, divided by height in inches again and multiply by 703

Obesity is defined by a BMI of 30 or more. Overweight is a BMI of 25-29.9. Normal weight is a BMI of 18.5-24.9. BMI has its limitations. Most importantly is, as stated, weight is made of more than fat. Fat is what we are concerned with for health implications. A bodybuilder will have a lot of weight but it may be mostly muscle. That person would still have a high BMI. BMI is also less accurate an indicator in the very tall and very short.

If you have a bio impedance/body composition scale you can get an estimate of your percent body fat. These scales are not very accurate in absolute numbers for body fat percent; however, they are useful to trend increases and decreases over time. Obesity is defined by a body fat percent more than 25% in men and more than 33% in women. This measure is limited in utility because it does not reflect the location of fat. Fat in the belly (i.e. intra-abdominal fat) is the type that is worrisome and associated with health risk. Fat in the butt, hips and thighs is less well correlated with poor health outcomes.

Waist circumference is a good indicator of abdominal obesity. More than 40 inches in men and more than 35 inches in women confers high risk for health problems. A good rule of thumb is to keep your waist circumference less than half your height. Your waist is measured above your hip bones, level with your belly button all the way around your body with a flexible soft measuring tape.

Waist to hip ratio is a good indicator of abdominal obesity. Calculated as waist circumference in inches / hip circumference in inches (waist in inches divided by hip in inches). Waist circumference measurement is described above. Hip circumference is measured all the way around at the widest location. For both measurements be sure to keep the measuring tap level. 0.86 or more confers high risk for health problem in women. 1 or more confers high risk in men.

Excess body weight, more specifically excess body fat is very concerning. It is associated with so many health issues. Here are some heath issues associated with obesity:

All-cause mortality (death for any reason)

Hypertension (high blood pressure)

High cholesterol (bad cholesterol)

Diabetes (sugar)

Cancer

Coronary Artery Disease (heart disease)

Stroke

Sleep Apnea

Arthritis (wear and tear on joints)

And so much more

There are also less physical consequences of obesity like:

Depression

Anxiety

Other Mental Health Disorders

Low quality of Life

The good news is a little bit of weight loss goes a long way. Just a 5% weight loss can make a huge impact. A weight loss of just 5% eases the burden on your knees and lower back, reduces breast cancer risk, reduces diabetes risk, reduces triglycerides (fat in your blood), lowers blood pressure and so much more.

You do not have to target a BMI less than 30 or reach a certain number to experience health benefits and improve your health from fat loss. Everyone will not be skinny and everyone does not desire to be skinny. However, we should all want to be our healthier version. A little weight loss can go a long way toward your "why." It's a journey. It's your journey. It's your destination. Small changes make big success. There is no need to rock your world, unless you want to.

Considerations to get you thinking:

1. What benefits can I expect with weight loss?

2. What can I expect to happen if I remain the same weight or gain weight?

3. What method will I use to track my weight loss progress?

Chapter 4

You've Got To Eat Something!

It can be really hard to even know where to start! Everyone has an opinion. Everyone claims scientific evidence, though everyone cannot show you the study. Everyone is an expert. It is surprising that with all of this know-how we are still an overweight society. The keto camp, paleo camp, zone camp, etc. all claim to have "the answer." The truth is there is more than one way to do most things. As you read in Chapter 1, we all have different goals. We differ in what we find acceptable, what we want for ourselves, effort we want to give, tolerance for progress and lack of progress, etc. I'm not here to tell you to eat this diet or that diet. I want to give you some facts to "chew on." You decide for yourself what you want to do. It's all about you.

The Basics

All of the energy in food comes from carbohydrate, protein and fat. No one class of energy is bad. Carbs (short for carbohydrates) are not bad. Protein is not bad. Fat is not bad. We need them all.

The energy in food is measured in calories. When weight loss is the goal we want to be mindful of the calories we eat. Eating more calories than we use to power our bodies' activities on a regular basis will result in weight gain. Except in athletes, for the average person this weight gain is in the form of fat.

Generally speaking, moderately active women should consume about 2000 calories per day and moderately active men should consume about 2600 calories per day for weight maintenance. Moderately active means a lifestyle of about 1.5-3 miles daily walking at a 3-4 mph pace in addition to light physical activities associated with daily living. Cycling, badminton, dancing, shooting baskets, walking golf, raking and table tennis are other activities with the same energy expenditure. The minimum calories needed to maintain body functions and weight is 10-15 calories per pound for the moderately active person. So, a 150 pound person would eat 1500-2250 calories daily to maintain.

Fat

The general recommendation for diet content is 20-30% fat, with less than 10% of this coming from saturated fat. Fat is the most calorically dense of all the energy sources. That means, if you have the same weight of fat, protein or carbohydrate…fat will have the most calories. It will actually have more than double the calories. Fat is 9 calories per gram. It just makes sense from a weight loss perspective to keep fat low in the diet. Fat calories not used for body's current need are stored on the body as fat.

We need some fat in our diet. However, the need is minimal. Vegetables and fruits contain minimal amounts of fat, with rare exception like avocado. For the most part the fat in plants (vegetables, fruits, beans and peas, nuts and seeds and whole grains) is helpful. They contain mostly unsaturated fat (coconut being an exception). Unsaturated fat can help lessen cardiovascular disease when it is replacing saturated fat.

Saturated fat is found mostly in animal meat and animal products, like dairy. It is also found in tropical oils like coconut and palm. It is a significant health issue. Saturated fat worsens cardiovascular disease (diseases of the heart and blood vessels).

Trans fats are the absolute worst for health. Artificial trans fats have been banned in the USA due to being unsafe. To avoid artificial trans fats still in food you must avoid hydrogenated or partially hydrogenated oils. The hydrogenation process creates trans fats. Hydrogenated oils can be found in shortening, some microwave popcorn, some margarine and vegetable oils, fried fast foods, bakery products, non-dairy creamer and processed foods. Equally dangerous, trans fats still occur naturally in dairy products and meat.

At 120 calories for just 1 tablespoon of oil, it is best avoided when planning for weight loss. Calories are better spent elsewhere because oil is not very filling. For that 1 tablespoon of olive oil at 120 calories, you could eat 30 olives … which do you think is more filling? Oils are a very calorie dense product with only a very small fraction of the nutrition contained in the whole food source.

Consider these low fat swaps:

Instead of donuts, muffins or croissants consider whole grain bread slice, whole grain tortilla or ½ bagel.

Instead of buttered, cheese or fried vegetables consider raw or steamed vegetables with spices.

Instead of full fat milk and cheese consider skim or 1% fat or low- fat yogurt.

Instead of bacon, sausage or hotdogs consider 2-3 ounces of lean meat, no skin on poultry, tuna in water, beans and peas.

Instead of mayonnaise, butter or cream cheese consider low fat versions or hummus.

Instead of fried chips consider pretzels.

Instead of any fried food consider baked or water/broth sauteed.

Carbohydrates

45-65% of our calories should come from this category. Carbohydrates are 4 calories per gram. They are less than half the calorie density of fat. Carbohydrates are our bodies' preferred energy source. The body can use fat and protein for energy but it is very inefficient and comes with sacrifice. Having carbohydrates in your diet is essential to burn fat, as desired with weight loss.

Carbohydrates are categorized as sugars, starches and fiber. They are found in grains (bread, pasta, crackers, and cereal), beans and peas, snack and cakes, juice and soda and veggies to name some. In general, we want to avoid added sugar, major in fiber, and eat some starch for optimal weight and health.

Simple sugars added to foods can be called raw sugar, brown sugar, corn syrup, high fructose corn syrup, glucose, fructose, sucrose and fruit juice concentrate to name some. They should be avoided when possible. Added sugar adds empty calories, meaning they add calories with no health benefit. Many foods, like fruit, naturally contain sugar. The sugar found naturally in whole foods is not an issue because it is packaged with fiber which slows absorption and has many health benefits.

All plants (vegetables, fruit, beans and peas, nuts and seeds and whole grains) contain fiber. Fiber makes up their structure. There is no fiber in animal products. A high fiber diet helps reduce cardiovascular disease, reduces cancer and promotes weight loss just to name some of the benefits. Good sources of fiber include barley, oatmeal, beans, nuts, apples, berries, pears, whole grains, carrots, greens and popcorn. If you buy a packaged food you want the carbohydrate to fiber ratio to be 5 or less, indicating it is a high fiber food. Current recommendations are 25-38 grams of fiber daily. Fiber should be the star and focus of your meal. Salads and wraps are good ways to get a lot of fiber in a low calorie meal. It is easy to load up on cooked and/or raw vegetables and greens in a salad or wrap. Be careful not to add too many nuts because they are calorically dense. Use fat free dressings or better yet, the juice from the fresh fruit on your salad. Consider fat free hummus instead of mayonnaise in your wraps. The extra bonus with fiber is that we do not digest it. Our bacteria digest soluble fiber to the tune of us absorbing about 2 calories per gram. Insoluble fiber does not count toward calories at all. Fiber should be the nutrient we are all gunning for.

Starches include foods like potatoes, corn, pasta, rice, bread, cereals and squash to name some. Starches are satiating, they help you feel full. They contain an abundance of nutrients.

Protein

Let's start by understanding, generally speaking, there is no protein deficiency in the developed world. We have been taught that high protein is needed to lose weight, we must eat meat and eggs or we must drink protein shakes. Nothing could be further from the truth. Here is where the confusion comes in, with significant weight loss you will lose both fat and muscle. We only want to lose fat, so in that case you should eat "enough" protein to support your musculature. Excess protein consumed and not used is broken down and made into sugar.

The general recommendation for diet content is 10-35% protein. Protein is also 4 calories per gram which is less than half the calorie density of fat. All meat, seafood and dairy products contain protein. However, it is packaged with harmful saturated fat. All plants also contain protein. The protein in plants is not the same as protein in animals. It is important to eat a wide variety of plant foods if this is your exclusive source of protein. Plant sources of high protein include beans and peas, nuts and whole grains. Soy milk is an easy swap for dairy milk with similar protein content.

Whole Foods

As much as possible eat foods in their natural form- the way they came out of the ground or off of the tree or vine. Processing, strips foods of their nutrients. It removes fiber and often adds sugar, fat and chemicals to preserve shelf life. These foods are often packaged and convenient but they promote obesity and make weight loss more difficult. Processed meats are classified (by the International Agency for Research on Cancer) as carcinogens, which means they cause cancer. Processed meats include- hotdogs, ham, bacon, sausage and some deli meats. They are in the same category as tobacco smoke. Red meat is classified as a probable carcinogen.

Liquid Calories Count

I recommend you avoid sweetened drinks. Be sure what you drink is providing nutrition, if it has calories. The best drink is water of course. Water which has no calories hydrates, lubricates, helps with bowel movements and reduces the calorie density of foods. If you cannot fathom the idea of drinking plain water, eat food with a high water content like- watermelon, strawberries, cantaloupe, peaches, oranges, cucumbers, zucchini, celery, tomatoes and peppers just to name some. These foods have high water content, low calorie density, lots of nutrients and fiber. You can also consider infusing your water with fruit and vegetables for added flavor. Cucumber mint infused water is particularly refreshing. We can sometimes mistake thirst for hunger. It's always good to start with water.

I recommend you avoid or at least limit juice, even 100% juice. Unfortunately, juice is really concentrated fruit sugar and water. The fiber has been removed. Some nutrients are present. I recommend eating the whole fruit so you get that perfectly packaged water, nutrient density, fiber and natural sugar balancing out.

Coffee and tea have some health benefits and may support weight loss. Be careful about adding sweeteners, creams and syrups which pack in calories. Excess caffeine can be harmful.

Smoothies can be a good way to get a lot of nutrients. They are a good way to get greens if you have trouble eating them. Be sure to have vegetables and fruit in your smoothie. You can use additional water if needed. It is not necessary to add milk, juice or yogurt to make a yummy drink. You should not put more food in your blender than you could eat in a meal. Try to make the smoothie last at least 20 minutes. Sipping instead of gulping and prolonging your intake allows time for the gut to signal the brain to slow your eating. It may be helpful and healthful to leave your smoothie a little chunky to chew a bit.

Sauces can add so many calories. Try to get in the habit of adding spices and herbs for flavor. Regular salad dressings and gravies can easily provide more calories than the food it is being applied to. Fat free dressings and tomato/broth based sauces are a better choice for weight loss.

Broth based soups are an excellent choice. Broth is low in calories being mostly water. You can fill your soup with plenty of beans, veggies and starches. We naturally eat soup slowly which allows the gut and brain to connect and reduce eating.

Alcohol is 7 calories per gram. It's almost double the calories for the same weight of carbohydrates or protein. It can contribute substantially to weight gain. Alcohol also inhibits fat breakdown which hinders weight loss effort. To top it off we often mix alcohol with sweetened drinks which adds to the calorie burden.

This chapter, like the others, is to share facts. There is no one size fits all, no perfect diet and you do not have to be 100% compliant with whatever diet you choose to experience benefits.

Considerations to get you thinking:

1. How will I reduce saturated fat in my diet?

2. How will I increase fiber in my diet?

3. How will I limit unhealthy liquid calories in my diet?

Chapter 5

Who Has Time For That?

In Chapter 4 we mentioned the "c" word, CALORIES. Now, I really don't want you to focus on that. I definitely don't want you to plan on calorie counting as a long- term plan for weight loss. It's important to understand the caloric contribution of the foods you choose. It's important to know how far off you may be from a goal. However, for most of us daily calorie counting is not a sustainable long-term plan. I recommend you track your calories initially to get an idea of what you have been consuming and to maybe learn tweaks that may work for you and how it may impact your overall intake. After you get an idea try to live based on whatever goals you set. If you find you aren't losing weight you can always adjust plan or track your calories again temporarily to figure out where you can improve.

There are so many calorie trackers available now. So many apps that are free. My favorite is My Fitness Pal. I think it is easy to use and has a robust data base. It also allows you to track your macros (percent fat, carbohydrate and protein). Myplate.gov is a helpful site that can be used to help you visualize and plan healthy meals. It also has an associated app.

You may already know you have a problem with portion sizes. It may be enough for you to eat on a saucer instead of a plate. Don't allow seconds, unless it's fruit or vegetables or after a certain amount of time has passed and you are still hungry. It's a worthwhile experiment to learn the difference between your portion size and a serving size. A serving size is generally written on a packaged food (serving size is not so much an issue with whole foods because you will generally be full before you eat too much) or can be found online for unpackaged foods like meat. You may discover the portion size you take in your meal is often 2-3 times the recommended serving size.

Intermittent fasting may appeal to you. This is the idea of an extreme reduction in food consumption for set periods of time. Some will fast every other day or so many days per week. Under this umbrella is also time restricted eating. This is the idea of eating only during a defined time period and fasting the rest of the day. This works best when you stop eating when the sun goes down. The period of not eating allows for bowel rest and can be healthful hormonally and for your gut microbiome. There are intermittent fasting apps to help keep you on target and find a community of like minded people. My favorite app for intermittent fasting is called LIFE.

Remember whatever change you make is a lifestyle change not a diet. Ideally a lifestyle change is set for a lifetime.

More than tracking calories, it is important to figure out how you want to live and what you want to accomplish. How can nutrition help or hurt you with that? One way to look at this is with food journaling. Food journaling is something else you may only do for a while to identify opportunities for improvement, opportunities for planning and awareness. It can be pictures of your meals on your phone, taking notes of what you've eaten, a spread sheet, app tracker, etc. It's important to include what times you eat, where are you, what are you feeling and how is the food prepared……. not just what you eat and the quantity. The more you record, the better your reflection and chance of making meaningful identifications. Here you can learn what works well and not so well for you. Journaling may help you identify triggers. Visual, auditory or olfactory ques that make you want to eat, even when you're not hungry.

Another approach is to focus on making "good food choices" instead of avoiding "bad food choices". In other words, crowd out the bad. Hold yourself accountable to what you decide is best for yourself. However; you must be flexible and adjust what works and does not work. Learn from your prior successes and failures. It may be a good idea to focus on changing your behavior and not so much your weight.

Since 1981 we have heard about SMART goals. This acronym first used in an issue of *Management Review* (Doran, G.T. (1981) There's a S.M.A.R.T. Way to Write Management's Goals and Objectives. Management Review, 70, 35-36), is helpful criteria for making goals that are attainable in a chosen time period.

S specific

M measurable

A achievable

R relevant

T time bound

SMART goals help us to be true to our plan by helping us think through, be detailed, know when we have succeeded and adjust as we go.

Weight loss is a journey. It's a very specific journey. It's very personal on every level. Like any journey it will not be a straight line. There will be ups and downs along the way. If you mess up in aligning with your goals just do better the next meal (don't wait until the next day). All is not lost. You learned from that experience.

Considerations to get you thinking:

1. How will I easily track my food intake?

2. What triggers me to eat when I'm not hungry?

3. What successful changes have I made in the past (not food)? What contributed to my success?

Chapter 6

Have A Notion For Motion

Activity matters. All activity matters.

Activity indicates energy expenditure or calories burned. Calories are burned with exercise and without exercise. Just existing burns calories and moving burns more. Non exercise activity thermogenesis (NEAT) is a term used to describe the energy used for activities other than sleeping, eating and exercise. NEAT includes standing, walking to the bathroom, climbing the stairs at work, chewing gum, fidgeting, typing, etc. NEAT is energy used in our day in and day out activities that are not planned exercise. It can account for a substantial number of calories daily. For example, a 102 calorie sitting hour at work can be a 174 calorie hour if standing. It varies from one person to the next and within an individual from day to day. It is highly modifiable. This is why steps walked can be thought of as an achievement, even if not steps done as part of a walking exercise program. Just move more. 10,000 steps daily is a nice goal and associated with health benefits. However, start any where and increase from there.

Ways to increase your NEAT:

Park further

Stairs instead of elevator/escalator

Standing/walking desk

Pace while on the phone

Walk to the desk of a co-worker instead of emailing or calling

Get stuff instead of sending your children to do it

Have a walking meeting

Use the bathroom on another floor

Actively play

Sweep instead of vacuum

Wash dishes instead of using the dishwasher

Choose an active job

Set a move alarm

Thermic Effect of Food

This is not a voluntary activity per se, but it's useful to understand and something we can influence. The thermic effect of food is calories burned from eating, digesting and otherwise processing food consumed. It amounts to about 10 percent of our daily energy expenditure. High fiber and protein rich foods have the highest thermic effect. Fat on the other hand is very easily processed and has very little thermic effect which is undesirable for weight loss.

Resting Metabolic Rate

This is our major energy expenditure, 70% daily. It is the energy used at rest, just existing. It can be influenced by choices we make. Too low of a calorie intake will lower your resting metabolic rate (RMR). Increasing muscle mass (not necessarily bulking up) increases RMR because muscle burns more calories than fat. Drinking cold water, tea, spicey foods, coffee and good sleep may all promote an increase in RMR, even if temporarily.

Exercise

Exercise is an obvious way to burn calories. I saved it for last in this module because I want to emphasize that it is highly recommended but not necessary for weight loss. Exercise should be thought of more for health benefits than weight loss in the average person. Think about this- walking 1 mile in 15-20 minutes may burn about 100 calories. 1 pound of fat is 3500 calories. So for this example, it would take 35 miles or 525-700 minutes to burn 1 pound of fat. Don't get me wrong, the benefits of exercise are undeniable and absolutely worth the effort, but I do not want to mislead anyone into believing it will account for the greatest impact on weight loss. Physical activity accounts for 15-20% of daily energy expenditure in the average moderately active person.

Benefits of exercise include improvements in:

Strength

Bone density

Aerobic capacity

Flexibility

Balance

Mental ability

Quality sleep

Sexuality

Benefits of exercise include reductions in:

Heart disease

Disability

Blood pressure

Cholesterol

Injury

Depression and anxiety

The recommendation for health is 150 minutes of aerobic exercise divided through the week. Aerobic activities include swimming, walking, running, cycling, hiking, jumping rope, dancing, etc. You will want to work at a pace that gets your heart beating faster than usual. Most people can do at least low impact, low intensity exercise like walking, water aerobics or exercise cycling.

Additionally, resistance or strength training is recommended. Resistance exercises include free weights, medicine balls, weight machines, resistance bands or even your own body. The general recommendation is to exercise each muscle group at least 2 times weekly on non-consecutive days. Each exercise should be repeated 8-12 times (called repetitions) in 2-4 blocks (called sets).

Exercise also increases energy expenditure when the activity itself is over. This bonus, called excess postexercise oxygen consumption, is higher for maximal strength training compared to modest aerobic activity.

Motivation

Besides your drive to reach your goals and live the life you want to have, you may require some physical motivation. Here are some ways to get the juices flowing to exercise when you feel less than excited:

Take a buddy

Listen to music

Listen to an audiobook

Listen to a podcast

Exercise in a different place or room

Go to a different gym

Try a different class or video online

Is It Safe

If you are unsure if you should exercise definitely **talk with your family doctor first**. Here are questions from a survey called Physical Activity Readiness Questionnaire (PAR-Q) used to identify people who should have medical clearance prior to starting exercise (Warburton DE, Jamnik VK, Bredin SS, et al. Evidence-based risk assessment and recommendations for physical activity clearance: An introduction. Appl Physiol Nutr Metab. 2011;36 Suppl 1:S1-2. doi: 10.1139/h11-060).

1. Has your doctor ever said that you have a heart condition and that you should only do physical activity recommended by a doctor?

2. Do you feel pain in your chest when you do physical activity?

3. In the past month, have you had chest pain when you were not doing physical activity?

4. Do you lose your balance because of dizziness or do you ever lose consciousness?

5. Do you have a bone or joint problem that could be made worse by a change in your physical activity?

6. Is your doctor currently prescribing drugs (for example, water pills) for your blood pressure or heart condition?

7. Do you know of any other reason why you should not do physical activity?

A "yes" to any question, even just one question means you should definitely talk with your family doctor prior to starting an exercise program. If you answered no to all questions it is reasonable to start slow and build up your exercise capacity. **However, I recommend you speak with your family doctor first anyways to be on the safe side.**

Considerations to get you thinking:

1. How will I increase NEAT?

2. How will I get my 150 minutes of weekly aerobic exercise? Keep in mind 10 minutes increments is fine.

3. How will I increase my motivation to be more active?

Chapter 7

How Do You Use Food?

I know that sounds like a crazy question. How do I use food? Who uses food? We eat food and make food… but use food? We can read all the way back to the bible days when Jacob used a bowl of stew to take Esau's birthright. He used food. It is important to understand how we use food if we are to control our intake.

Much of our food use is social. We go out for drinks or coffee. We party with food. We mourn with food. We connect over a meal. We use it as a symbol of connection. We have emotions associated with these events and it underscores the consumption. Good conversation, presents and activities, expressive words and hugs and so much more could give these events as much meaning if not more.

Some of us eat because we are bored. We want some stimulation. We want our senses to be moved and excited. We want to feel something, when we otherwise feel numb. We may find food comforting. After a long and hard day, having a familiar meal that is associated with good comforting emotions is quite inviting.

We may use food to influence or as a means of demonstrating effort or love. We have all heard the saying, "the way to a man's heart is through his stomach."

Historically food has been associated with status. There is something to be said for being able to afford to go to "nice" restaurants with white table cloths and high prices to eat "rich foods."

We use food for reward. Who has never said to yourself, "I deserve a treat for xyz? This one time won't hurt." Often times whatever we accomplished that provokes that thought is a reward in itself.

Some may find safety in food. They think if everything else is out of control and crazy and I don't have anything else, I know I can eat.

Some may find protection in food. Food supplies energy for weight. Their body weight, their mass, may be used for intimidation. It may be intricately tied to how they see their strength (even when it is fat mass and not muscle mass). It may feel like a security blanket in this way.

Some may use excess weight, and the food that fuels it, for attention. The attention may be good or bad. For some, women especially, it may protect from unwanted sexual attention. For some, it may attract the attention of just the type of wholesome person they want, someone undeterred by excess body fat because of the greater value of a person.

Some use food for fuel. To fuel the activity of the body. To be in optimal shape. To function at the top of their abilities. To fight off diseases and prevent other diseases.

The idea of mindfulness is ancient but became more of a mainstream psychologic tool around the 1970s. At the heart of the concept is being present in every moment. In this application it is being attune to your food intake.

Eating when you are hungry, slowly enough to taste each flavor and how it mixes, appreciating texture, consider what nutrition is being provided and do so undistracted (especially by a screen). Mindful eating may help you uncover how you use food.

There is no right or wrong here. No judgment to be made. There is only insight to be had. Understanding how we use food will help us understand our own motivations and drives which will inform our goals.

Considerations to get you thinking:

1. How do I use food? Is it appropriate and healthful? If not, what will I do about it?

2. How will I express social connection without including food?

3. How will I reward myself without including food?

Chapter 8

Planning is Everything

Have you ever heard Benjamin Franklin's quote, "If you fail to plan, you are planning to fail." It is so true. It is a rare thing for someone to stumble upon success. Having a plan that becomes your routine is optimal. Routines do not take up much mental space. Here, I am going to suggest some planning and routines for you to consider in your weight loss journey.

Plan your meals in advance. Plan all of your meals including your snacks. Meal planning and prepping help you to always have a nutritious option available. Choosing something else would require more time, more money and/or more effort. Hopefully in that time and space you will make the more healthful choice that supports your weight loss goals. If you don't want to prepare all of your meals and snacks for the week at one time then have a plan for when you will fit it in. There are degrees to meal preparation and planning. Consider slicing and dicing produce when you get home from the store, portion size food in bags, label meals, portion out meals, cook and freeze meals, get lunch bags ready, etc. You make it as thorough as it needs to be for your success. Even if you are not going to prepare your own meals, meal planning is essential. Consider a meal delivery service that will prepare meals aligned with your goals. Then you only need to plan for snacks. At the very least have a daily plan for what you will eat and how you will obtain it easily in your day, and have a healthful back up plan.

Grocery shop with a list. Try to stick to your list. Concentrate on the periphery of the grocery store. You will find your vegetables, fruits, nuts/seeds, meat and fish all on the periphery. Go down the aisles only if you need to and get only what you need for your planned meals and snacks. Go to the grocery store after eating a meal. Don't go when you feel stressed or tired. If you don't want to eat something, don't buy it. Junk food isn't healthful for anyone so it doesn't need to be in your home. Your children, partner or anyone else in your home can benefit from a kitchen with only healthy foods. If you are going to purchase a junk food item, never buy the family sized bag.

Try to make a habit of making your first meal of the day your heaviest meal with progressively smaller meals to a light dinner. Our bodies process calories differently depending on what time of the day we eat. It is helpful to have time to move around and do something with the calories we consume before laying down for the night.

Try to be consistent with where you eat in your home. It will help with mindfulness. Perhaps you decide to only eat in the kitchen at the table… which means you would not eat at the counter in a rush or in front of the TV mindlessly. Be mindful of your triggers. Move trigger items out of site and put desirable items in plain view.

Plan ahead when you eat out. Check out the menu online. Look for healthful options or substitutes and low calorie dips and sauces. Ask for your meal to be prepared without butter or oil. Don't upsize. Have a salad or broth-based soup prior to your entrée or as your entrée. Drink water. Dilute sweetened drinks with water. Take half of the meal home or share a meal. Eat before you go to events where food is served that may not align with your goals. Take a low-calorie dish to a potluck and eat it first. Stand far from high calorie food trays at events.

As with most things a good plan is a great start. Getting into a routine is extremely helpful for this weight loss journey. This is not a diet you go on and go off. This journey will be long lasting so a good plan you can make routine will be so valuable and lessen your perceived effort over time.

Considerations to get you thinking:

1. How will I plan and prep my meals?

2. What impediments can I anticipate and how will I get ahead of them?

3. What healthy meals will I have at my usual restaurants?

Chapter 9

Stress Less And Rest Well

Stress

Stress less is so much easier said than done. It's necessary on this journey to weight loss. For some of us this will be the hardest part. Our perception of stress has such broad manifestations throughout our bodies. It impacts the way we function, perceive, respond and even the way we present ourselves to others. There are so many sources of stress which contributes to our difficulty with managing it. We can feel overwhelmed in our relationships with significant others, children, family care, work, health, finances etc. The list of sources of stress goes on and on. The need for management is crucial.

Stress increases cortisol levels in the body. Cortisol is critical to survival. However, when chronically elevated it can be harmful. Chronically high cortisol promotes weight gain and fat deposition, especially abdominally. Elevated cortisol levels also increases food cravings and appetite.

Stress can be managed if we learn to own our thoughts. Thoughts may pop up in our minds but we do not have to allow them to settle there. We can train and retrain our minds to combat negative thoughts with positive thoughts. We can train and retrain our minds to not ruminate on what is not in our control. Think of the time you can give back to your life if you repurpose time you spend stressing.

It can be helpful to have a support group or 2 or 3. Sometimes a vent session is all you need to free that space in your mind and move on. You must consider; however, you are venting to someone who may also need to vent. So instead of simply thanking them, you must listen as well. A support group that provides a degree of anonymity may be preferable. Therapy does not have the stigma it once had and more and more people see the value in seeking this assistance.

No. That is a complete sentence. We must learn to say it and feel comfortable with making our limitations known and respected. It can be a challenge initially, but it gets better with practice.

Sometimes it's necessary to change your environment. It's a good idea and always appropriate to evolve. If your evolution is helping you become more of who you want to be, then by all means stay, improve, take it like a champ and suck up those growing pains. However, there are times when you're in an environment that is changing you for the worse. It may be best then to change location.

Sleep

Sleep is important to restore your body for optimal performance. Sleep deprivation results in elevated cortisol levels with the deleterious effects mentioned earlier. Poor sleep results in increased hunger due to poor hormone signals and lower resting metabolic rate. Practically speaking not sleeping may lead to more snacking.

Having a good sleep routine to promote a restful night is a good idea on this journey. The following are ideas for sleeping well:

1. Have a set bed time and wake time

2. No caffeinated beverages in the evening

3. No screen time a couple hours prior to sleep and no screens in the bedroom

4. Don't nap during the day

5. Exercise regularly

6. Manage stress

Considerations to get you thinking:

1. What negative thoughts do I need to change?

2. What positive thoughts will I replace them with?

3. What/who do I need to say no to?

Chapter 10

Food Addiction

Food addiction is a real thing and is probably under diagnosed. It's truly beyond the scope of this book to get into it. However, I want to increase awareness. If you think you have food addiction please **discuss this with your family doctor** so that you can get the help you need. Like any other addiction, food addiction requires professional assistance from someone trained in the field.

The following questions are from the Modified Yale Addiction Scale Version 2.0 (https://pubmed.ncbi.nlm.nih.gov/26866783). The statements are related to the previous 12 month period. Scoring helps identify individuals who may suffer from food addiction.

1. I ate to the point that I felt physically ill.

2. I spent a lot of time feeling sluggish or tired from overeating.

3. I avoided work, school or social activities because I was afraid I would overeat there.

4. If I had emotional problems because I hadn't eaten certain foods, I would eat those foods to feel better.

5. My eating behavior caused me a lot of distress.

6. I had significant problems in my life because of food and eating. These may have been problems with daily routine, work, school, friends, family or health.

7. My overeating got in the way of me taking care of my family or doing household chores.

8. I kept eating the same way even though my eating caused emotional problems.

9. Eating the same amount of food did not give me as much enjoyment as it used to.

10. I had such strong urges to eat certain foods that I couldn't think of anything else.

11. I tried and failed to cut down or stop eating certain foods.

12. I was so distracted by eating that I could have been hurt (e.g. when driving a car, crossing the street, operating machinery)

13. My friends or family were worried about how much I overeat.

Joel Fuhrman offers this yes or no self- test for food addiction (*Fuhrman, Joel. (2015). The End of Dieting: How to Live for Life. HarperOne)*. With this test two yes answers confirm addiction to food and one yes is suspicious for addiction to food.

1. If I don't eat regularly, I feel fatigued or irritable.

2. I think about eating certain foods almost all the time.

3. I feel sluggish or uncomfortable after eating.

4. Eating poorly is interfering with my health.

5. I'm overweight, but I continue to overeat.

6. When I start eating sweets, I don't want to stop.

7. I have tried to diet to lose weight but failed and given up.

8. I prefer restaurants with all-you-can-eat buffets.

9. I have physical withdrawal symptoms.

10. I sneak food when others aren't around or looking.

11. I store food or hide food from my family.

12. I eat more even though I'm no longer hungry.

13. My eating habits cause me distress.

14. My eating habits are causing me social and family difficulties.

15. I eat almost continuously all day long.

Again, if you think you have food addiction please discuss this with your family doctor so that you can get the help you need.

Consideration to get you thinking:

1.   Is it possible I have food addiction?

52

Chapter 11

What Has Worked For Others?

The National Weight Control Registry follows over 10,000 people who have lost at least 30 pounds and kept it off for at least 1 year. Much can be learned from their efforts. The following was captured from their website (http://www.nwcr.ws/Research/default.htm):

> 98% of registry participants report that they modified their food intake in some way to lose weight.

> 94% increased their physical activity, with the most frequently reported form of activity being walking.

> Most maintain a low calorie, low fat diet and do high levels of activity.

> 78% eat breakfast every day.

> 75% weigh themselves at least once a week.

> 62% watch less than 10 hours of TV per week.

> 90% exercise, on average, about 1 hour per day.

A study (Kliemann N, Vickerstaff V, Croker H, Johnson F, Nazareth I, Beeken B. The role of self-regulatory skills and automaticity on the effectiveness of a brief weight loss habit-based intervention: secondary analysis of the 10 top tips randomised trial. International Journal of Behavioural Nutrition and Physical Activity. 2017, 14:119.)

of the habits of people who successfully lost weight and kept it off in the UK suggests the following:

Regular meal routine, meals at the same time daily with no snacking

Choose healthy fats

Aim for 10,000 steps daily

Pack healthy snacks when you go out

Always look at labels

Start w a glass of water, follow with smaller portions

Move more

Choose water, limit juice

Eat mindfully

Aim for five servings of vegetables daily.

This gives an idea of what has worked for others. I hope you have some ideas about what can work for you. Remember this is a journey with ups and downs. Your course is yours alone. A mess up does not mean throw in the towel. It's an opportunity to figure out what works and does not work and an opportunity to do better with the next meal. You determine your own goals, set your plan and make it a routine.

Remember your why. You will need to come back to it many times. It will be your driving force and help remind you of your destination.

Considerations to get you thinking:

1. What will I apply to my life from the registry participants?

2. What habits will I apply from the study participants who successfully kept weight off?

3. What is my why?

Conclusion

Thank you so much for lending your attention to *Weight Loss For Life For Regular People.* I hope you're taking some information with you that will change your life and help you become the best version of yourself.

Feel free to send a comment to allaboutyouwellness.net@gmail.com

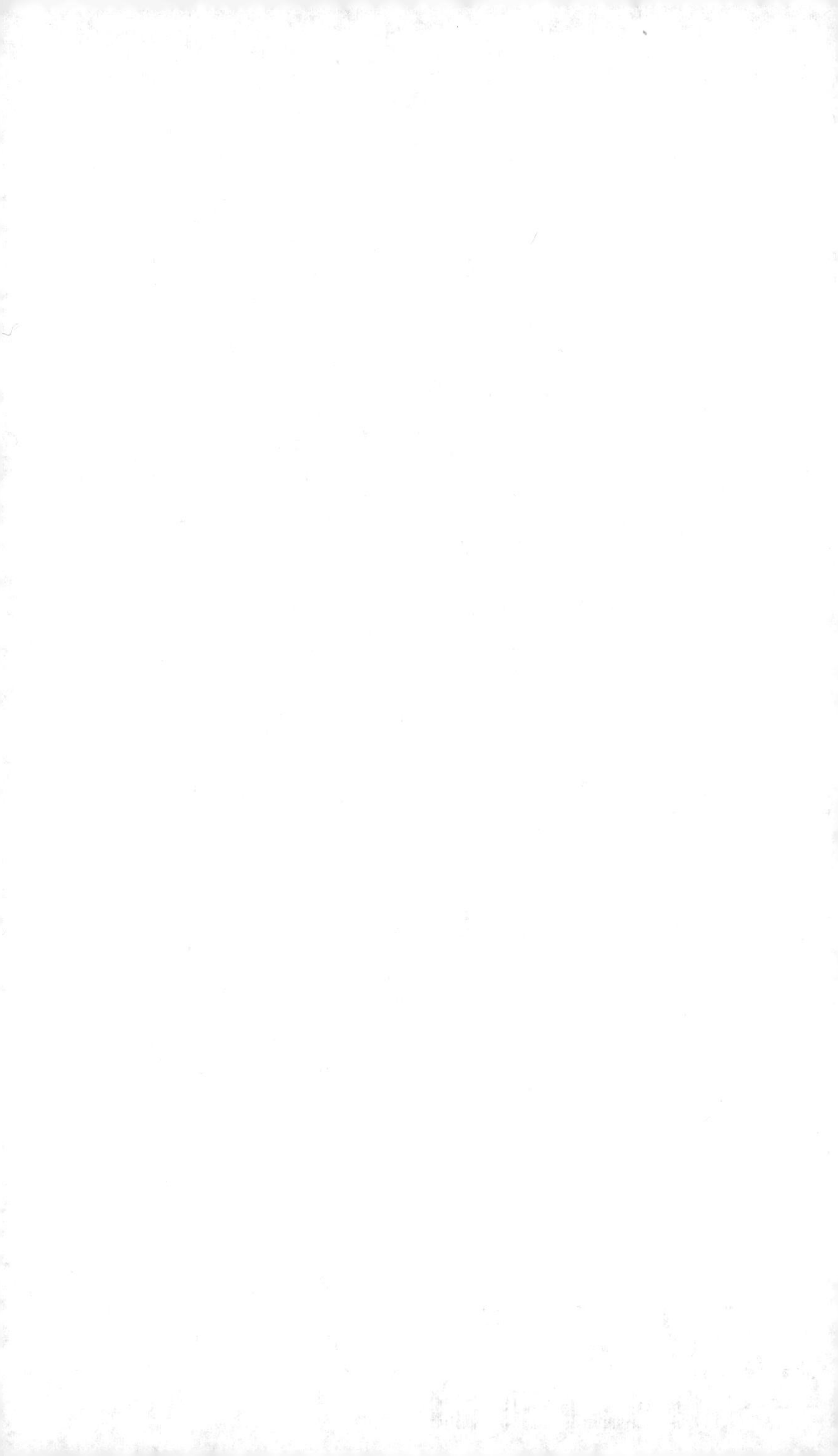